Nerve Mobilization
of The Upper Extremity

Dedicated to Wayne
who has always supported me...

Caroline Joy Co, PT, DPT, CHT, CSFA

Nerve Mobilization of the Upper Extremity

Rehabsurge, Inc.'s mission is to support healthcare and education professionals to continue their educational and professional development. Rehabsurge is committed to identifying, promoting, and implementing innovative continuing education activities that can increase and impart professional knowledge and skills through books, audiobooks, or digital e-books based on sound scientific and clinically derived research. The first Rehabsurge continuing education book was published in July 2009.

As a sponsor of Continuing Education (CE) seminars and workshops, we enable professionals to enhance their skills, pursue professional interests, and redefine their specialties within their respective disciplines while earning CEUs, CE credits, or Contact Hours. Offerings include CE books, audiobooks, and digital e-books, all of which are focused on the latest treatment and assessment approaches and include discussions of alternative and state-of-the art therapies.

Disability Policy:

Rehabsurge seeks to ensure that all students have access to its activities. To that end, it is committed to providing support services and assistance for equal access for learners with disabilities. Rehabsurge has a firm commitment to meeting the guidelines of the Americans with Disabilities Act and Section 504 of the Rehabilitation Act of 1973. Rehabsurge will provide support services and assistance for students with disabilities, including reasonable accommodations, modifications, and appropriate services to all learners with documented disabilities.

ISBN: 1449910637
EAN-13: 9781449910631
Printed in the United States of America

Disclaimer:

This book is intended for informational and educational purposes only. It is not meant to provide any medical advice.

For permissions and additional information contact us:

Rehabsurge, Inc.
Phone: +1 (516) 515-1267
PO Box 287
Email: ceu@rehabsurge.com
Baldwin, NY 11510.

About the Author

Caroline Joy Co, PT, DPT, CHT, CSFA, is a licensed physical therapist and certified hand therapist whose clinical experience includes acute, subacute, home health and outpatient settings. Her background includes Community Based Rehabilitation designed to assist people with disabilities access rehabilitation in their communities using predominantly local resources. She is the President and CEO of PTSponsor.com, an online resource for U.S. hospitals and clinics that seek to sponsor and hire foreign-trained physical therapists. She specializes in hand therapy through an integrated approach that includes education, counsel and exercise. She is also certified in functional assessment for work hardening and work conditioning.

Her background includes current employment with Better Healthcare Inc, Mercy Medical Center and Silvercrest Center for Nursing and Rehabilitation. Her past affiliations include Long Beach Medical Center, Horizon Health and Subacute Center, and Grandell Rehabilitation and Nursing Center.

She is a professional speaker for Summit Professional Education, Cross Country Education and Dogwood Institute for hand rehabilitation; myofascial release and nerve mobilization; coding, billing, documentation and ethics. She received her transitional doctorate from A.T. Still University and her BS in physical therapy from University of the Philippines-College of Allied Medical Professions. She is licensed in California, Nevada and New York.

Full Disclosure

To comply with professional boards/associations standards, all planners, speakers, and reviewers involved in the development of continuing education content are required to disclose their relevant financial relationships. An individual has a relevant financial relationship if he or she has a financial relationship in any amount occurring in the last 12 months, with any commercial interest whose products or services are discussed in their presentation content over which the individual has control. Relevant financial relationships must be disclosed to the audience.

As part of its accreditation with boards/associations, Rehabsurge, Inc. is required to "resolve" any reported conflicts of interest prior to the educational activity. The presentation will be scientifically balanced and free of commercial bias or influence.

To comply with professional boards/associations standards:

I declare that neither I nor my family has any financial relationship in any amount occurring in the last 12 months, with a commercial interest whose products or services are discussed in my presentation. Additionally, all planners involved do not have any financial relationship.

Caroline Joy Co, PT, DPT, CHT, CSFA

Course Description

Injuries to the peripheral nervous system often result in significant deterioration of the regular activities. Many of the peripheral nerve injuries in the upper extremity are commonly associated with altered shoulder postures and functional imbalance in the arm, forearm, and hand. It is essential to know about the basics of the nervous system, the neuropathology, the transmission of pain, and movement dysfunction before initiating nerve mobilization procedure. The movement of the nerves or nerve fibers can result in changes on the internal nerve physiology by altering the neural tension. Neural mobilization aims to relieve such changes in the nerve physiology to alleviate symptoms of pain and restriction of mobility. It is also vital to have a clear idea about the principles, guidelines, precautions, and contraindications of nerve mobilization for better utilization of this procedure.

Course Objectives

1. Implement techniques of Upper Limb Tension Testing (ULTT) to rule out proximal pathology from hand symptoms.

2. Apply nerve gliding and muscle re-education, in the treatment of common upper quadrant problems.

3. Design a home exercise program for the client with upper quadrant problems.

4. Describe the common entrapment sites and pain mechanisms in the cervical spine, shoulder, wrist and hand.

5. Identify the most common anatomical sites of upper extremity compression

6. Examine the neural system continuum and its relationship to musculoskeletal problems using Upper Limb Tension Testing (ULTT) to rule out proximal pathology from hand symptoms.

7. Demonstrate upper limb tension tests with a bias toward the median, ulnar and radial nerves.

8. Use proven techniques including neural milking, muscle stripping, nerve sliding and nerve tensioning to safely and effectively treat the median, ulnar and radial nerves.

Table of contents/Course Outline

CHAPTER 5   Treatment Techniques

CHAPTER 6   Review of Current Research and Concluding Remarks

CHAPTER 1

Anatomy and Physiology of The Nerves

Introduction

The nervous system is a complex arrangement of the nerve cells and tissues. It regulates the body responses to external and internal stimuli. The peripheral nervous system is responsible for the transfer of information between the motor and sensory neurons and their effectors in both directions.

Injuries to the peripheral nervous system often result in significant deterioration of regular activities. Many of the peripheral nerve injuries in the upper extremity are often a result of traction injury to the brachial plexus. Such injuries are commonly associated with altered shoulder postures and functional imbalance in the arm, forearm and hand due to pain in the related nerves and muscles. Brachial plexus neuropathy is one of the commonly noted upper extremity pain syndromes. The involvement of peripheral neuropathies and cervical spine pathologies can complicate the diagnosis of brachial plexus neuropathy.

The injury process of the nerves can be put into 4 stages: microtrauma, inflammation, scar formation and ischemia. These painful nerve lesions can become traction neuropathies and result in permanent/chronic disability of affected extremities if not diagnosed and treated early.

Most of the nerve injuries are believed to arise due to the influence of physical factors that alter the mechanical abilities of the nerve fibers. Nerve mobilization has been projected as an efficient therapy to treat the pathologies of the nervous system. It is essential to know about the basics of the nervous system, the neuropathology, the transmission of pain and movement dysfunction before initiating nerve mobilization procedure. The movements of the nerves or nerve fibers can result in changes in the internal nerve physiology by altering the neural tension. Neural mobilization aims at relieving such changes in the nerve physiology to relieve the symptoms of pain and restriction of mobility. It is also vital to have a clear idea about the principles, guidelines, precautions and contradictions of nerve mobilization for better utilization of this procedure (Ellis & Hing, 2008).

Importance of proper evaluation

Evaluation of the nerve injuries is as important as its treatment. Several conditions are often overlooked during the examination process which may result in incorrect diagnosis and inappropriate treatment. It is advisable to evaluate the musculoskeletal problem as well as the neurovascular problem in case of injuries. It is common to have a neural component associated with a musculoskeletal condition. The evaluation should be thorough and should include specific examinations to identify or rule out the possibility of any of the disorders. Once the correct diagnosis is made, the treatment protocols are decided.

Anatomy and physiology of the nerves

A basic understanding of the nerve structure and the initiation and transfer of pain impulses are necessary to evaluate the type and cause of neural pain and arrive at a conclusive diagnosis. A clear diagnosis of the underlying injury helps to form a proper treatment plan which would prevent the occurrence of complications.

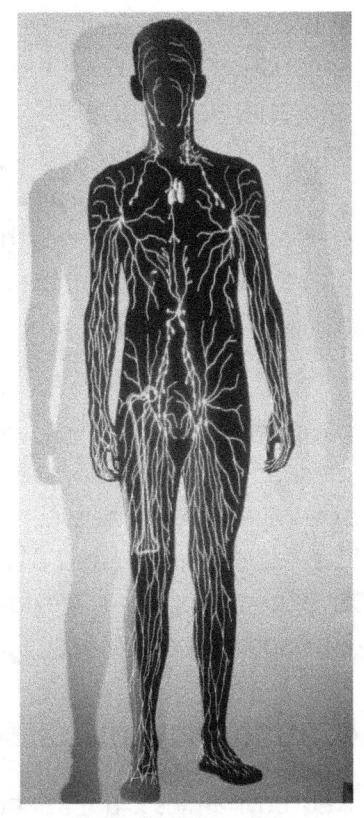

The nerve cells are composed of cell bodies and nerve fibers (in the form of axons and dendrites). The nerve fibers are arranged in bundles and are referred to as fascicles. Three layers of connective tissue cover the nerve fibers. They are the epineurium, perineurium, and the endoneurium. These connective tissue structures allow for gliding and sliding of the nerve. A nerve has to move according to the movements made by the body.

The endoneurium forms the initial covering of the nerve fibers after the myelin sheath. This layer also forms the interfascicular connective tissues. A bundle of individual nerve fibers each covered by a layer of endoneurium is known as the fascicles. The perineurium is a strong connective tissue structure that binds the fascicles. This perineurium controls the flow of fluids and ions in and out of the nerve cells and is a diffusion barrier to interfascicular fluid. It also assists in preventing nerve kinking at angles in response to compression forces. The epineurium forms the outermost covering that surrounds the nerve. It makes up the largest part of the peripheral nerve. The epineurium assists with interfascicular gliding to allow nerve elasticity or for the nerve to bend. It binds the fascicles and cushions the nerve from extraneural injury. It has a well-developed lymphatic channel but has no lymphatic vessels. The perineurium layer offers strength in tension. It also maintains the so-called blood-nerve barrier. The epineurium layer consists of areolar tissues that act as a cushion for the nerve fibers. This layer is highly vascular and is slightly coiled in order to adapt to the minor extension movements. The epineurial blood vessels have smaller branches that course all inner parts of the nerve (Bove, 2008).

The connective tissue sheath constitutes about fifty percent of the peripheral nerve. This structure helps the peripheral nerves handle mechanical forces more effectively. The amount of the connective tissue coverage ranges between 21% (as in the case of the ulnar nerve at the cubital tunnel) and 81% (as noted in the sciatic nerve). The fascicle arrangements allow flexible movements of the sensory, motor, and autonomic fibers (Millesi, Zoch, & Rath, 1998).

Neurodynamics

Neurodynamics is the science of the relationship between the mechanics and physiology of the nervous system. The nervous system starts with the brain and spinal cord and goes out to the peripheral nervous system that includes both somatic as well as autonomic nerves. The nervous system adapts to body movement in two ways. One is a sliding movement and the other is a rise in tension within the system (Pahor & Toppenberg, 1996; Wright, Glowczewski, Cowin, & Wheeler, 2005). Nerve mobilization causes decreased intraneural and extraneural pressure. It also improves blood circulation. A slider is a non aggressive movement which helps decrease anxiety in anxious patients. A tensioner is different from a slider because it is a more aggressive movement and it is applying tension from both ends (Wright et al., 2005).

It is vital for the nervous system to be able to adapt to changing mechanical loads. The nervous system undergoes many distinct mechanical events such as elongation, sliding, angulation, cross-sectional change, and compression (Ellis & Hing, 2008). The nervous system becomes vulnerable to conditions such as neural edema, fibrosis and ischemia if it is not able to adapt to the mechanical changes. Altered neurodynamics is often considered as the cause for many neural disorders that result in a significant amount of morbidity (Butler, 2000; Shacklock, 1995).

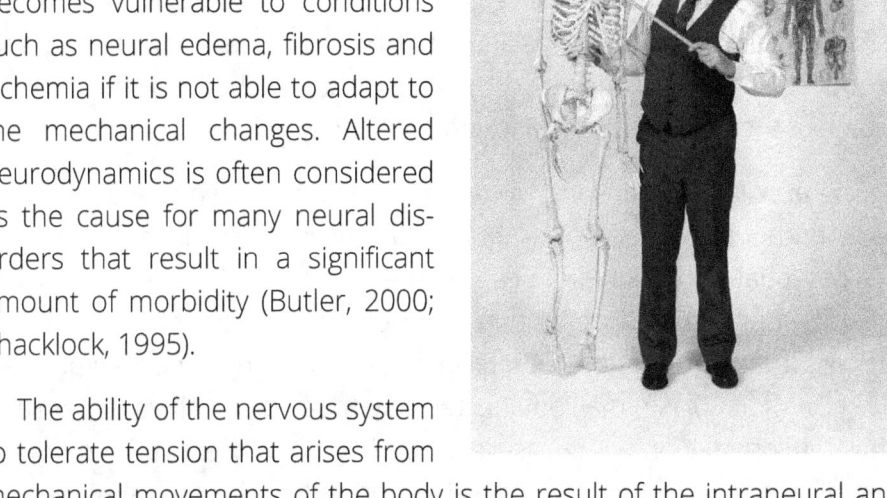

The ability of the nervous system to tolerate tension that arises from mechanical movements of the body is the result of the intraneural and extraneural architecture. The nerve is quite tortuous internally, which allows it to be stretched freely to a certain extent (Sunderland, 1965). Further movement is aided by the ability of the nerve fibers to undergo intraneural or extraneural gliding. This gliding motion helps in attenuation of the tension that arises from the movements of the body. Intraneural gliding is noted between an individual nerve fiber and the endoneurium. It is also noted between nerve fibers with endoneurium and between the fascicles. Extraneural gliding is noted between the perineurium and the epineurium (Sunderland, 1978; Millesi et al., 1990).

Common causes of reduced nerve gliding

The brachial plexus may be pinched due to an arthritic change or a first rib positioning variations. Arthritic joints may cause synovitis which can close the tunnel in the area through which the nerve is passing. Work-related upper limb disorder or repetitive stress injury can occur if one is working in the same position for a long period of time. This tends to create buildup of lactic acid that reduces the ability of the nerves to glide. Entrapment of the nerve can also occur due to positional default. Tenovaginitis (inflamed and thickened retinacular sheath) such as de Quervain's produces swelling and edema which reduces nerve gliding. With myofascial pain syndromes, a trigger point or a tight muscle can also reduce nerve gliding. Surgery produces a local inflammatory process that can hamper the smooth gliding of the nerve tissues (Mackinnon, 2002).

The axoplasmic transport system provides the nerve tissues with the basic nutrients and other essential substances. Normal transport of all the essential nutrients is critical for the health of a nerve. The flow of these essential substances within the axons is a constant and controlled process that is designed for efficient transmission of nerve impulses. The flow of axoplasm may be affected due to factors such as ischemia or physical constrictions. A pressure gradient generally exists in the nerve that allows the movement of blood in and out of the neural tissue. For optimal flow through the nerve tissues, the pressure in the artery must be greater than the pressure in the capillary, which in turn must be greater than the pressure in the neural tissue. Abnormally elevated pressure results in hypoxia that can lead to edema and fibrosis as a consequence of oxygen deficiency. On the other hand, reduced venous flow can also lead to hypoxic states and fibrosis due to pooling of blood for a prolonged period of time. This fibrosis stage can occur in a single fascicle or in multiple fascicles (Shacklock, 1995).

Maintenance of the pressure gradient across the nerve tissues and the blood vessels within the nerve tissues is vital for effective exchange of substances. Several factors can affect the pressure gradient being maintained at different interfaces (Shacklock, 1995). Physical force applied on a nerve due to an external or internal compression, ischemia in the nerve tissues that occurs due to factors such as tissue injuries, and postural demands from occupation around the nerves can bring about changes in the pressure gradient (Shacklock, 1995).

The blood supply to the nerve tissues can be altered by several factors among which compression has an important role. Research has shown that arterial blood supply is reduced even if the nerve tissue is stretched by only seven to eight percent of its overall length. Wright et al. (1996) studied cadavers to evaluate the ability of the nerves to move during body movement and strain. They noted that the median nerve slides two centimeters (about 35 mm) at the wrist from wrist extension to wrist flexion. They concluded that this sliding ability of the nerves allows us to perform the day to day activities that require different types of movements at the wrist joint (Turl & George, 1998). Another study by O'Driscoll et al (1991) evaluated the pressure at the cubital tunnel during movement and strains. It was then determined that the cubital tunnel is fifty percent smaller during flexion when compared to extension movement. Thereby, the cubital tunnel is open at extension, but as you go into flexion, it is fifty percent smaller. It was noted that the pressure in the cubital tunnel could go as high as 60mmHg which is significant.[18] Hence, when you have trauma to an ulnar nerve, it usually occurs with excessive flexion, excessive wrist extension as well as shoulder flexion for a long period of time. The inability of the nerves to glide can result in nerve compromise.

The severities of symptoms that may be noted depend on the duration of the compression, the severity of the compression as well as the number of sites compressed. Researchers have shown that factors related to intraneural movements, microcirculation and axon transport have a direct effect on physiological activity of a nerve tissue. Butler (1991) notes that with intraneural compromise, pain and symptoms that occur are just above the normal or stretch-like pain. Paresthesia is present. It is usually vascular in origin and it is instantly reversible with stopping of distortion. The extraneural nerve compromises, on the other hand, are associated with catching, twinging pain around vulnerable surfaces. The pain is intermittent and may be evoked by movement at interfaces. The symptoms tend to become severe with the increase in interface distortion (Butler, 1991). Mechanical interface is defined as the tissue or material adjacent to the nervous system that can move independently of the system (Butler, 1991; Turl & George, 1998; D'Mello & Dickenson, 2008).

The nociceptive afferent nerve fibers are capable of carrying noxious stimulation to the central nervous system and invoking the response in the form of pain. These nerve fibers are capable of sensing mechanical or thermal stimuli both externally (such as from the skin) and internally (from the muscles and organs). Afferent A delta and C fibers are the nociceptive afferent nerve fibers present in our body. These nerve fibers can be stimulated when exposed to mechanical forces, chemical irritants, or extreme temperatures. While the C fibers can be stimulated by processes such as edema and stiffness, both A-delta and C fibers are responsive to inflammation (Messlinger, 1997).

> ### POINTS TO PONDER
>
> *If I have a patient that has neuropathic pain, why can't a conduction study or an EMG pick this up? EMG or nerve conduction velocity tests one nerve at a time. The neuropathy may be in only one fascicle or the problem may be in connective tissue, not the fascicle.*

Pain Responses and Definitions

Nociceptive pain is generally considered to be the pain mediated by a noxious stimulus to a structure that is innervated by the nociceptors. A common example to explain this phenomenon is the immediate pain experienced when one hits their hand to any object accidently. The mechanical pressing of the hand tissues is the noxious stimuli sensed by the nociceptors present in that part of the hand. This is converted into electrical impulse and conducted to the central nervous system to generate the perception of pain (Bove, 2008; Robinson & Gerbhart, 2008). Peripherally evoked neurogenic pain originates in the nerve tissues outside the dorsal horn of the spinal cord. The presence of an abnormal impulse generating site for pain leads to non-painful stimuli being perceived as painful. An example of this would be a complex regional pain syndrome patient who has allodynia wherein the non-painful stimuli is perceived as painful. If you have an abnormal impulse generating site, the stimuli can be perceived as painful.

Allodynia refers to the condition where pain is felt from stimuli that do not hurt in normal circumstances. There are three types of stimuli that can cause allodynia-- mechanical forces, irritating chemicals and adverse temperatures. Anesthesia means loss of sensation commonly perceived as numbness in the affected regions. Hyperpathia refers to the increased pain response to a painful stimulus. The perceived pain may also continue to increase following the cessation of stimuli, but it does not continue for long periods of time (Butler, 1991). The nociceptive pain is generally related to mechanosensitivity and also with C-fiber impulse generation process. This type of pain has memory wherein the same non-painful stimulus can evoke pain on repeated occasions (Chen, 2008; Marchettini, Lacerenza, Mauri, & Marangoni, 2006).

Nerve Injuries Classification

The classification of peripheral nerve injuries was initially proposed by Seddon in 1942 and was converted into a more detailed classification by Sunderland in 1951 (Butler, 1991; Butler, 2000). Proper understanding of the type of nerve injury is essential to form the treatment plan.

Butler (2000) proposed that physical therapists should be able to identify and interpret the following categories of peripheral nerve injuries: 30the potential lesion; physiological pain; the inflamed and irritated nerve (irritation within the epineurium, and breach of the perineurium); and fibrosis of varying degrees (intraneural and extraneural). Butler (2000) suggested that the categorization of the peripheral nerve injury must be based on the symptoms, physical signs and their relationship.

Knowledge about nerve pathology must form the basic cue that drives the categorization.

Sunderland (1961)	Seddon (1942)	Injury	Recovery Potential
I	Neuropraxia	Intrafascicular edema, conduction block; Possible segemental demyelination	Full (1 day to 2 months)
II	Axonotmesis	Anatomic disruption of axon with little disruption of connective tissue; Axon severed; Endoneurial tube remains intact	Full (2 to 4 months)
III	Axonotmesis	Endoneurial tube torn	Slow; incomplete (12 months)
IV	Axonotmesis	Only epineurium intact	Neuroma-in-continuity
V	Neurotmesis	Anatomic disruption of axaon and connective tissue; loss of continuity	None
VI	Neurotmesis	Combination of above	Unpredictable

Stevens (1934) has laid down three important rules to be remembered while diagnosing a patient with nerve injury in the upper extremity.He suggests that the brachial plexus is injured either at its roots beyond their exit from the spine and before they join with other roots to form the plexus (trunks) OR in the terminal branches of the arm. The plexiform part of the brachial plexus is never injured except by cuts or wounds. However, it may get involved secondarily to hemorrhage and accumulation of exudates between the nerve bundles (Stevens, 1934). Tension and gliding of the nerve tissues has been noted to occur within the confines of the musculoskeletal system in response to the combination of certain specific body movements (Wilgis & Murphy, 1986).

The nerve mediated signs and symptoms can be initiated or exacerbated if a nerve or nerve root that moves with normal functional body movements becomes affected. Inflammation or damage of the nerve tissues by chemical mediators, macroscopic or microscopic trauma or entrapment of the nerve can result in such reactions. Such conditions are often associated with the appearance of pain (Butler & Jones, 1991; Elvey, 1986; Millesi et al, 1998; Bove, 2008) Pathological changes in the extra and intraneural anatomy may be noted in response to chronic repetitive compression or traction. Such nerve injuries are associated with paresthesias, motor weakness and altered deep tendon reflexes (Butler & Jones, 1991; Wilgis & Murphy, 1986; Walsh, 2005). Neural tension testing can be a valuable clinical test to help in the differentiation between neural and non-neural anatomic structures (Butler & Jones, 1991; Millesi et al., 1998; Butler, 2000).

CHAPTER 2

Evaluation Using Neural Tension Tests

Neural tension tests, also referred to as neurodynamic tests, are often employed by physical therapists and other healthcare providers to differentiate between the pathoanatomic structures responsible for pain. These tests are often employed to diagnose the cause of pain in the neck and lower back regions (Davis et al., 2008; Rubenstein & van Tulder, 2008). Some of the commonly used neural tension tests (NTTs) include the straight leg raise test (SLR), seated slump test (SST), and upper limb tension tests (ULTT).

The advancement of neural tension testing has been credited to researchers such as Butler (1991), Elvey (1986), Shacklock (2005), and Maitland (1985). The following sections will describe in detail the slump test and the upper limb neural tension tests.

These tests can be used to assess the active motion dysfunction and the passive motion abnormalities. Care should be taken to identify the presence of encountered resistance (such as reflex contraction of the muscles) and the irritability (patient response). This helps in preventing the progression beyond the end point of resistance and symptoms. The symptoms may be exacerbated if any movement is attempted beyond the end points (Davis et al., 2008).

Slump Test

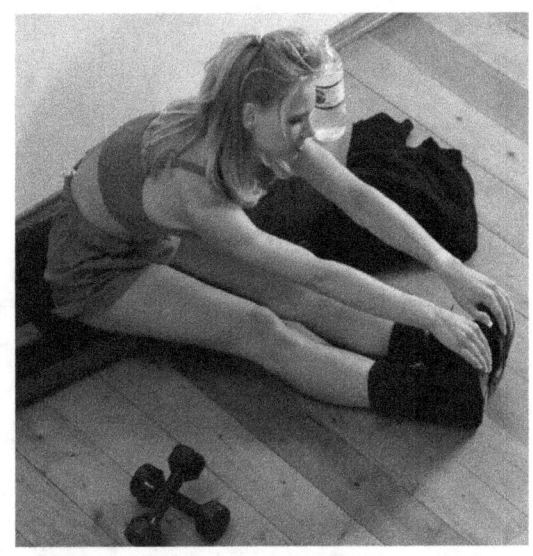

The slump test also known as the seated slump test (SST) actually came in existence in 1909 and was used from 1909 until 1970 when Maitland (1991), an orthopedic physical therapist, developed a modified slump test which was used for spinal problems. The slump test is performed by stabilizing the pelvis, flexing the head and moving a limb (Elvey, 1986; Maitland, 1985). Neural reaction will show the specific nerve in the lower extremities involved.

After the slump test was used and found reliable, the upper limb tension test was developed. Elvey (1986), another Australian physical therapist, wrote about the brachial plexus tension test in 1979. This upper quadrant nerve test was able to bring on signs and symptoms of the three major nerves in the upper extremity. In 1991, Butler continued to work on his upper limb tension testing by provocation of symptoms.

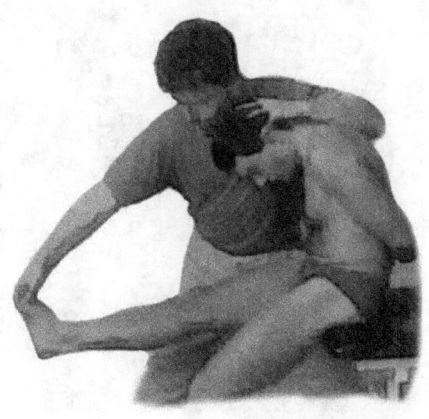

The slump test is believed to help in the evaluation of the sensitivity of neural structures such as the meningeal tissues, nerve roots, and the sciatic and tibial nerves (Magee, 2002; Maitland, 1985). A change in the symptoms and range of motion, resistance to extension of the cervical spine and reproduction of the symptoms are required to claim the test to be positive (Shacklock, 1995; Kleinrensink et al., 2000).

Upper Limb Tension Test

The upper limb tension test (ULTT) differentiates symptoms arising from neural tissue and from non-neural tissue. The range of motion of the joints must be tested first as the interfaces may be limited. A test is positive when there is a reproduction of symptoms. Adverse neural dynamics happens when tightness in a muscle causes compression of the nerve, resulting in nerve entrapment. This can also lead to a decrease in the movement in the nervous system, as the forces are not dispersed. Further, an increase in the mechanical forces is also noted. Development of scar tissue may be initiated due to decreased dispersal of surrounding irritating chemicals (Millesi et al., 1990; Pahor & Toppenberg, 1996; Rozmaryn et al., 1998; Coppieters, Stappaerts, Eveaert, & Staes, 2001).

The major sensitizing movements are called biases. Start actively. Have the individual move actively before passive testing. Test the noninvolved extremity and then test the involved extremity. The ULTT consists of a combination of movements such as scapular depression, shoulder abduction and external rotation, elbow extension, forearm supination, wrist and finger extension, and contralateral cervical flexion (Butler & Jones, 1991; Butler & Gifford, 1989). This test is considered positive when there is a production of neural-mediated symptoms during elbow extension, and reduction of

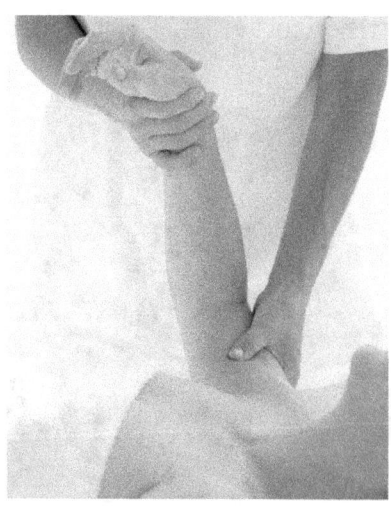

symptoms or an increase in elbow extension when the cervical spine is laterally flexed toward the involved extremity (Butler & Jones, 1991; Davis et al., 2008).

The sensitizing test in ULTT is cervical lateral flexion away from the symptomatic side. If there is pain, you can bend the neck away towards the asymptomatic side to make sure that you use the entire neck for testing.

Soft tissue mobilization may be needed in such cases to ensure that the joint is moving properly. The radius and ulna should also be evaluated for their gliding ability. Exercises are prescribed for a few weeks. Retesting for presence or relief of symptoms must be performed after a suitable interval period.

There are three ways to depress the shoulder girdle. The first way is to just depress the shoulder girdle. The second way is manually cupping the hand over the scapula and then depressing the shoulder girdle. The third way is gently pulling down on the arm. When you perform shoulder girdle depression and reproduce the symptoms, then, you know that the cause of the symptoms is proximal. It may be the cervical area or it may be the brachial plexus at the shoulder region.

A patient comes to you in a protective posture. The protective posture is when the patient holds the painful arm towards the chest. The head is slightly tilted to the painful side. This patient has pain with full elbow extension and while moving the wrist from flexion to extension.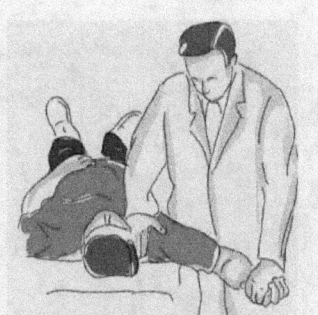

If lateral flexing of the head to the non-painful side reproduces the symptoms, the connection is from the central nervous system to the peripheral nervous system. The cause is proximal.

Next, move the patient into some degree of shoulder abduction then wrist extension. As symptoms decrease, move the head to the non-painful side. Side-bending to the non-painful side can relieve the symptoms, while elongation of the nerve occurs by side-bending to the opposite side. Work the patient through by doing repetitions. This involves performing multiple repetitions of general elongation, general sliding, and gliding of the nerve.

You can reproduce the pain in symptomatic patients by compromising the median nerve in this test. Check for trapping of the nerve, muscle tightness, trigger points and correct them appropriately with nerve gliding and muscle stretching. Remember to support the arm well while performing these techniques.

Make sure that it is not a faulty breathing pattern that has compromised the neck and upper extremity. The patient should relax by using abdominal breathing as opposed to scalene or upper trapezius breathing. Look for shoulder movement when the patient is breathing. Make sure that the scalenes do not entrap the nerve. Start by performing strengthening exercises for the diaphragm. The glenohumeral abduction is a sensitizing movement that can be related to C5, C6, or C7 nerve root, wherein the nerve may be pulled from the foramen. It may be related to brachial plexus not sliding properly between the pectoralis minor and coracoid process. In this case, if there is a true muscular tightness, ways to stretch these muscles need to be followed. If glenohumeral abduction is the sensitizing movement, a normal response would be no pain or very slight paresthesia, but a

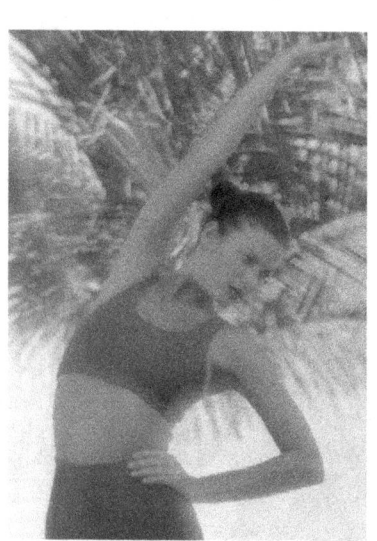

positive response would be tightness in the anterior aspect of the axilla as well as with slight paresthesia in the shoulder.

If you have someone that has an irritable nerve, it is obvious that you just do not want to go in and stretch the individual too quickly. Test actively first!

Therefore, if the muscle tightness is causing the compromise, you not only have to move the joint, you should also stretch the tight muscle and make sure that the connective tissue is moving so that the nerve can move properly.

What about lateral flexion? We know that, with the head in neutral position or side bent toward the painful side, it takes the some of the stretch away from the nerve. With contralateral side flexion, slack is taken out from the nerve root. Tension is built in the scalenes. The normal response may be moderate pain and limitation of movement. A positive response would be decreased range of motion and an increase in symptoms (Kleinrensink et al., 2000).

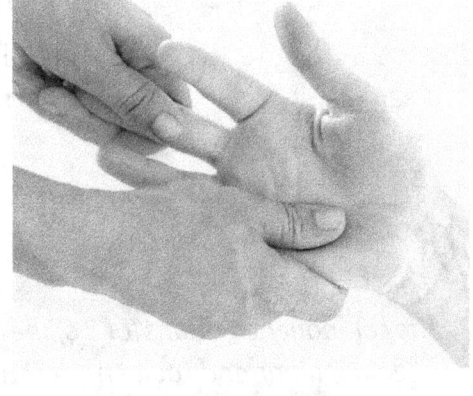

By extending the neck you unload a portion of the nerve. If you choose to extend the neck, it unloads the dura. The slider position is assumed by putting the head in extension, because it unloads the neck. If you have the shoulder girdle depressed and cervical spine flexed, you load both ends of the nerve. The tensioner position is assumed by putting the cervical spine in flexion, because it loads the neck and the upper extremity.

Signs and Symptoms

The signs and symptoms vary based on the condition.

Normal

Deep ache or stretch in the cubital fossa, anterior and radial aspect of the forearm, radial aspect of hand, anterior shoulder area, and tingling to the finger. These symptoms increase with contralateral cervical flexion and decrease with ipsilateral side flexion.

Pathological

1. Reproduction of patient's symptoms.

2. A sensitizing test in the ipsilateral quadrant alters the symptoms. For example, in testing the median nerve, wrist flexion increases elbow extension.

3. There are different symptoms between the right and left upper extremity (Butler, 1991).

The component motions for 3 of the major nerves in the upper extremity (median, ulnar and radial nerves) are detailed in the table on the next page.

Although the order of these components may be varied, testing each nerve in the standard manner is recommended.

Radial Nerve	Shoulder abduction Shoulder internal rotation Pronation Wrist/thumb-index flexion Elbow extension Shoulder depression Cervical contralateral flexion
Median Nerve	Shoulder abduction Shoulder external rotation Forearm supination Wrist/finger extension Elbow extension Shoulder depression Cervical contralateral lateral flexion
Ulnar Nerve	Shoulder abduction Shoulder external rotation Pronation or supination Wrist/small finger extension Elbow flexion Shoulder depression Cervical contralateral lateral flexion

CHAPTER 3

The Three Main Nerves of The Upper Extremity

Median Nerve

The median nerve is formed by the median and lateral cords of the brachial plexus from C5, C6, C7, C8 to T1. Test the median nerve when a patient presents thenar muscle, wrist and finger flexor weakness and sensory disturbances.

The palpable areas for the median nerve would be the upper arm medial to the biceps tendon, indirectly at the carpal tunnel which is between the palmaris longus and the flexor carpi radialis, and in the brachial plexus.

Areas of Entrapment

1. Test for pronator teres syndrome (entrapment at the ulnar and humeral head of the pronator teres): have your patient flex the elbow at 90 degrees, fully supinate the forearm. The therapist will resist coming into pronation.

2. Test for median nerve entrapment at the biceps area: resist flexion and supination of the forearm. This maneuver entraps the median nerve at its fibrous band and lacertus fibrosus.

3. Test for entrapment under the fibrous arch of the flexor digitorum superficialis muscle: Hold the patient's elbow in extension and resist proximal interphalangeal (PIP) flexion of the third digit.

Median Nerve Active Test

At the starting position, the arms are going to be at the side. Ask the patient to abduct the arms, externally rotate the shoulder, supinate, and extend the elbow. Then, extend the wrist and finally side-bend the head away from the painful side. If side bending the head causes symptoms, then the cause is proximal. Bring the head back to neutral and ask them to do wrist extension only; if this brings about symptoms, then, the cause is distal. A positive active quick test happens when there is a neurogenic change to the median nerve. The upper limb tension test for the median nerve will duplicate an ache or stretch at the cubital fossa over the anterior lateral aspect of the forearm and hand, and tingling in the thumb and index finger. There should be a reproduction of symptoms.

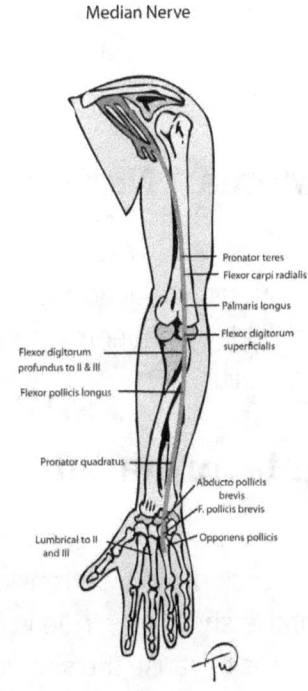

Median Nerve

Median Nerve Passive Test (High arm abduction)

Ask the patient to keep the shoulder girdle in slight depression and then move into shoulder girdle abduction; followed by forearm supination, wrist and finger extension, shoulder girdle external rotation, and elbow extension. If you are not able to elicit any pain, then, evaluate the proximal segment. This is accomplished by lateral flexion away from the painful side. As you abduct the limb, you work from 80 to 110 degrees. You will not be able to achieve this range if there is anterior wall chest tightness. The second thing you should do after shoulder abduction is wrist extension. After wrist extension, do forearm supination. The next movement is shoulder external rotation followed by elbow extension. If the symptoms have not been reproduced, contralateral cervical flexion can increase symptoms. Whatever test position you start, whether it is distal or proximal, you have to follow the exact sequence. This helps you design the best treatment program.

Median Nerve: low abduction

This is done exactly like the standard high abduction test. However, shoulder abduction is only performed at 20-30 degrees. This is suitable for elderly patients and patients with dislocatable shoulder or adhesive capsulitis.

Interpretations

If you note that components such as median nerve abduction, wrist extension, elbow extension, and supination are not painful, but depression of the shoulder girdle is painful, it suggests brachial plexus compression. This is because the shoulder girdle depression catches the brachial plexus between the clavicle and first rib. A positive response would be noted, if there was a brachial plexus entrapment injury proximally with the median nerve. There would be pain in the neck and top of the shoulder with slight paresthesia as you depress the clavicle on the first rib.

When you do wrist extension, anatomically, nerve gliding occurs on both the median and ulnar nerves. If the flexor retinaculum tightens, the pressure in the carpal tunnel increases. Extending the fingers and thumb, allows the flexor tendon to move approximately by 2 to 3 cm. This causes an increase in the median nerve pressure. Our normal response with wrist extension would be just a general stretch pain at the wrist but a positive response would be more than a stretch pain, it would be paresthesia.

Ulnar Nerve

The ulnar nerve travels with the brachial plexus. It pierces the intermuscular septum between the flexors and the triceps muscles. It travels along the triceps muscle to pass under the ulnar collateral ligament, which runs between the humerus and the ulna. Then, it passes underneath the flexor carpi ulnaris. Finally, it travels between the flexor carpi ulnaris and flexor digitorum profundus and superficialis. It reappears at the wrist just slightly on the radial side of flexor carpi ulnaris tendon. The sensory division continues out to innervate the hypothenar side of the hand and the last two fingers.

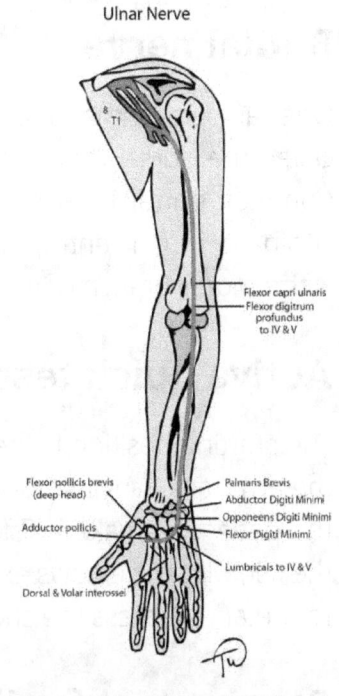

Ulnar Nerve

The ulnar nerve comes from the medial cord of the brachial plexus, C8 to T1. It is palpable at the pisiform at the wrist as well as the cubital tunnel at the elbow. Those are the two common entrapment areas of the ulnar nerve.

If you have ulnar nerve injury, you might be positive for a Froment's Sign.

A Froment's Sign is dysfunction of the adductor pollicis. If you hold a piece of paper, you substitute the motion by flexing the interphalangeal joint because the adductor is weak.

Active quick test for the ulnar nerve

In the active quick test for the ulnar nerve, the patient can be sitting or standing. Ask the patient to put the hand on the ear while the fingers are pointing upwards. Then, ask the patient to turn their fingers down toward the shoulder. This is an active quick test to evaluate the irritability or the amount of pain associated with the ulnar nerve.

Radial nerve

One can palpate the radial nerve at the mid humerus. The sensory division called the dorsal radial sensory branch is also palpable at the forearm. Common entrapment syndromes could be de Quervain's tenosynovitis, supinator muscle entrapment and the posterior interosseous nerve which is the motor branch of the radial nerve at the forearm.

Active quick test with the radial nerve

The starting position is the patient standing while the arms are hanging down by the side. Then, ask the patient to make a fist with the thumb inside the fist, with the elbows extended. Then, internally rotate and depress the shoulder girdle.

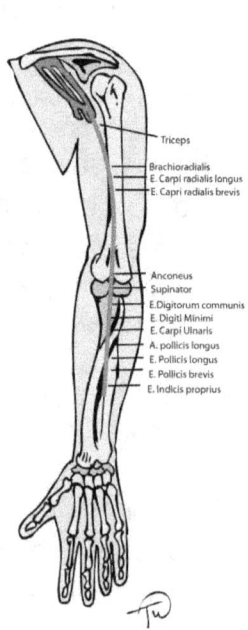

Radial Nerve

Triceps
Brachioradialis
E. Carpi radialis longus
E. Capri radialis brevis

Anconeus
Supinator
E.Digitorum communis
E. Digiti Minimi
E. Carpi Ulnaris
A. pollicis longus
E. Pollicis longus
E. Pollicis brevis
E. Indicis proprius

Passive test for the radial nerve

The passive test for the radial nerve is begun with the patient in supine position. The patient's shoulder needs to be slightly over the edge of the bed. The therapist depresses the shoulder girdle. Then, the next step is elbow extension which is followed by shoulder internal rotation and forearm pronation. Wrist and thumb flexion can be added for further sensitivity.

CHAPTER 4

Exercises To Improve Nerve Gliding

Median Nerve Exercises

Balloon patting exercise

This exercise is done with a balloon. Pat the balloon from one hand to the other hand. This exercise should be performed gently.

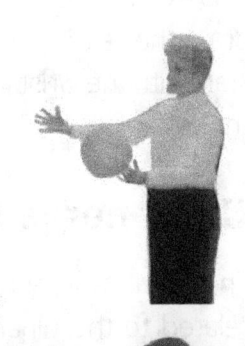

Wrist stretch

The wrist is in flexion and then you use the other hand to extend it. Use the noninvolved limb to put a stretch on the involved side. So, if there was a right median nerve problem you would use your left hand to push your right wrist up into extension and do resistive exercises in that position. If it is painful, you could start with an elbow flexed position.

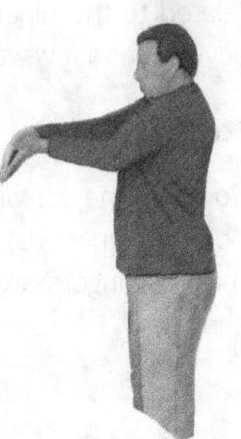

Crawling exercises

Position the patient in crawling position. Progress by asking the patient to flex the neck.

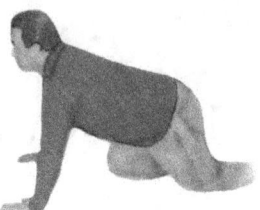 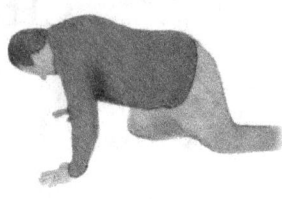

Alphabet letters

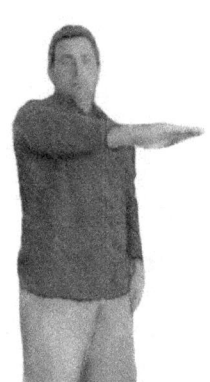

This technique is a simple exercise wherein you draw the letters in the air with the hand. You can start with the wrist in neutral. Progress by extending the wrist.

Ulnar nerve exercises

There are several types of home exercises prescribed for relieving pain related to the ulnar nerve. These are simple to perform and are to be advised for a few weeks.

I can't hear you

Cover up the ear with one hand (with the fingers pointing upwards), then rotate the hand so that the fingers are pointing down towards the shoulder.

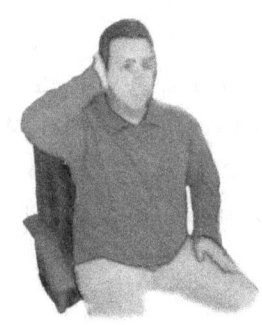

Avoid the glare

Cover the face gently with the elbow flexed. This is similar to covering your eyes to avoid the glare from the sun.

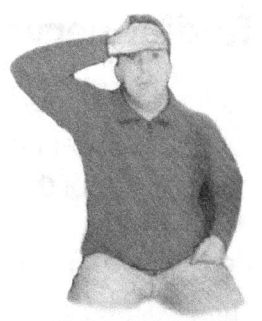

Plate carrying technique

This is an exercise where one imagines carrying a plate in the hand. The individual loads the elbow, puts the wrist in extension and starts from shoulder elevation and abduction. Shoulder depression may be added to progress this exercise.

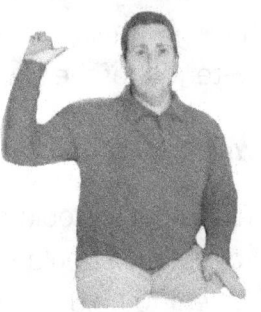

Towel Exercises

You take a towel and dry the back and then you switch arms.

Sunglasses and spiderman

Make an "O" with your fingers, place the "O" directly around the corners of your eyes. This is the sunglasses position. If you are flexible, you can reverse the sunglasses. This is what we call the spiderman position. The long, ring and little fingers should be pointing to your chin.

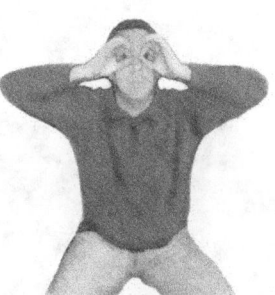

Radial nerve exercises

There are several self-management strategies that can be advised for the management of pain and other symptoms associated with the radial nerve. Some of these have been listed below.

Pouring water

The exercise involves holding a cup upright and then internally rotating it so as to mimic pouring water out of the cup.

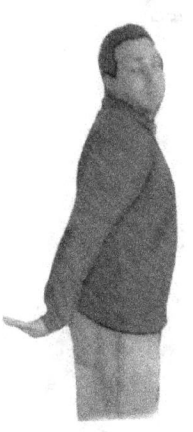

Waiter's tip

The patient should put the hand behind the back, so that the shoulder is in internal rotation. Ask the patient to hold out with the thumb flexed and the wrist flexed.

CHAPTER 5

Treatment Techniques

The patient must be educated about the role of the nerves in the occurrence of symptoms and should be made aware how the modulation of the nerves assists in relieving the symptoms. The therapist must have a thorough knowledge about the anatomy and physiology of the nerves in question.

The treatment must be chosen based on the presenting problem and must take into consideration all the applied aspects of the nerve pathology. It must be individualized for each patient. Finally, the therapist must encourage the patient to perform the home care measures. Periodic follow-through to evaluate the progress and to advise changes in the exercise protocols are also equally important. The treatment is generally advised in three stages.

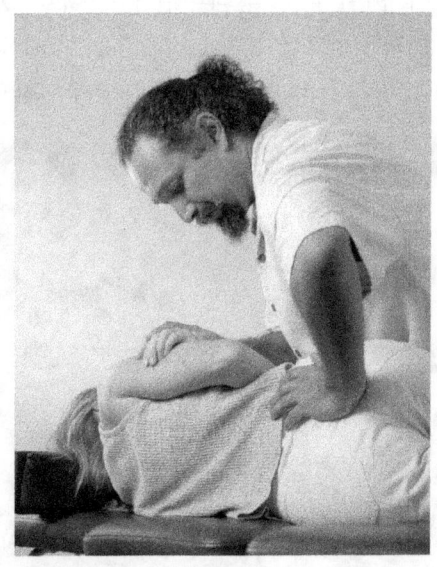

Stage I – Symptom Control

The first stage involves making appropriate changes in the behavior of the patient to bring about relief from constant traumatic practices. Certain changes at home and workplace are advised to relieve the tension in the affected regions. Relieving tension reduces constant pressure on the nerves and muscles and decreases the frequency and the severity of the symptoms. Some of the methods used to control the symptoms have been listed below:

Behavior modification

The patient should be asked to bring about certain modifications in everyday activities. The main idea is to create awareness about the need for these changes so that the patient can change his practices that may be causing the injury. Care should be taken to address the active myofascial trigger points. Pain modulation through different modalities and exercise should be considered. Some of the steps that you can advise your patient to follow include appropriate positioning of the upper extremity (UE) at rest to avoid placing tension on the nerve; avoid exertional breathing or increased exertional activity ; wearing padding that increases surface pressure from automobile shoulder restraint straps; wearing a strapless bra and avoid carrying heavy objects.

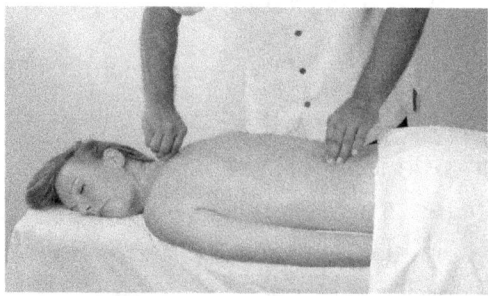

Minor modifications in the regular activities can significantly relieve the muscle and nerve tension and bring about symptom relief. Some modifications include resting the extremity on the arm rest of a chair/ pillow (30 min before sleeping); placing hand in coat pocket, and proper sleep positioning.

The subconscious stretching of the muscles and nerves can worsen the symptoms or affect the prognosis of the treatment. The sleep position must be evaluated and the patient must be provided with guidance about proper sleep positions. The patient must be encouraged to maintain the spine in neutral position while sleeping. Care should also be taken by the patient to support the upper extremities in a position without tension while sleeping.

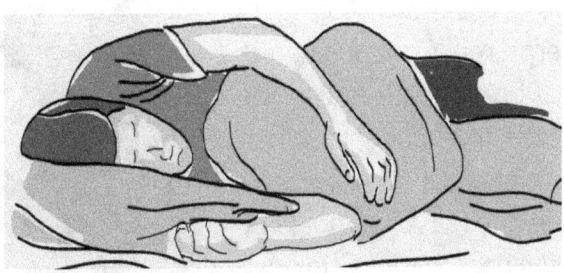

Workplace modification

Many individuals suffer from nerve entrapment due to improper posture assumed at the workplace. While exercises and nerve gliding can relieve the entrapment, workplace modifications must be advised to hasten the recovery time and prevent the recurrence of the symptoms. Improper postures such as keeping the head forward with rounded shoulder while working in front of a computer for long duration can exert undue pressure

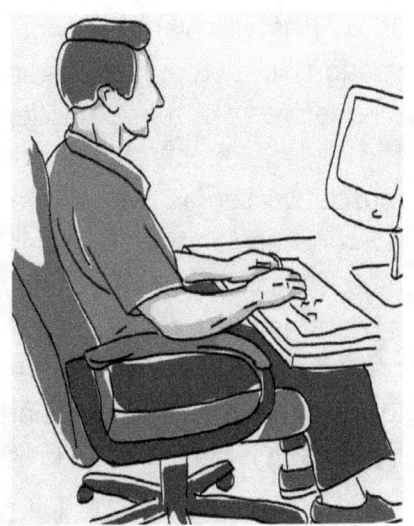

on the shoulder. The head should be held straight in line with the back and the shoulders must be in a straight and comfortable position. The patient must also be advised to limit overhead positions of the upper extremities.

Breathing Pattern

Breathing techniques need to be modified to bring about relief from neural tension and pain. A low impact, tolerable aerobic program must be advised to encourage large segmental muscle group activity. Accessory breathing patterns must be eliminated. Diaphragmatic breathing must be demonstrated to the patient. When you have a tight cervical or any upper quadrant muscle, the nerve cannot glide easily The nerve has to slide through a scar linkage which causes it to be pinched and swollen. Muscle tightness is

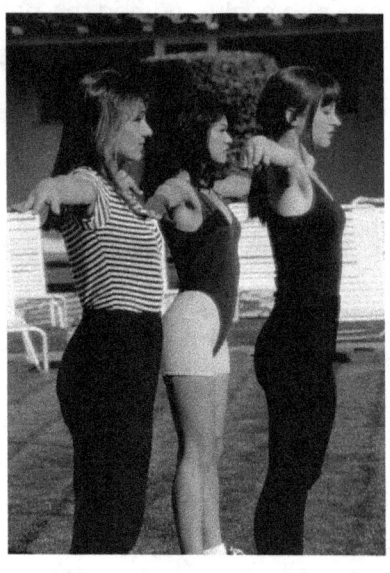

associated with joint stress, soft tissue dysfunction, neural compromise as well as vascular and lymphatic compromise. There is a functional relationship between the agonist and antagonist muscle. If you have a muscle spasm or tense muscle, it can inhibit the antagonist muscle which can lead to a double cross syndrome. The rhomboid and serratus anterior muscle weaken as the pectoral muscles as well as upper trapezius and levator scapulae muscle are all tight. Posture plays an important part in muscle weakness or muscle imbalance. A forward head posture leads to a shortened serratus anterior muscle and a lengthened middle and lower trapezius muscle. The scapula becomes abducted which increases the load on the glenohumeral joint. Chronic nerve compression can result if the muscle is tight and the pressure within the muscles is increased.

Stage II – Restorative Procedures

The restorative procedures can be initiated once the symptoms have been reduced. Initiation of these procedures before the symptoms have been reduced can make it difficult to mobilize the nerves and muscles effectively. The restorative procedures involve many important steps. These include manual techniques such as mobilization of the soft tissues and joints, deep massage and stretch, nerve gliding, and home exercises. Home exercises help in improving the flexibility of the muscles and the nerves and prevents the recurrence of the symptoms. These exercises also help in strengthening the muscles to a certain extent. Manual techniques that involve massage and stretching are performed to improve flexibility, restore normal tissue lengths, and restore normal posture. These techniques may be repeated if required.

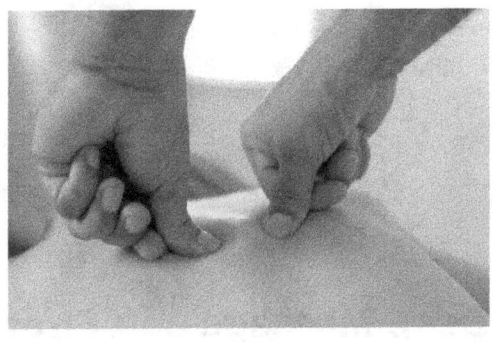

Soft Tissue Mobilization/ Muscle Stripping

The soft tissue mobilization procedure involves stretching, applying deep pressure and traction. The purpose of this method is to move the tissue fluids, relax the muscles under tension and release the trapped layers of connective tissue (fascia) that are creating bodily dysfunction. Mobilize the acromioclavicular and sternoclavicular tissues. Perform muscle stripping on the muscles that can potentially compress on the nerve such as the pronator teres for the median nerve, flexor carpi ulnaris for the ulnar nerve, supinator and brachioradialis for the radial nerve. Muscle stripping is using the fingertips, the ulnar border of the hand (little finger side), the thumb or the elbow to apply pressure along the muscle fibers usually from origin of the muscle to insertion.

Joint Mobilization

The mobilization of the affected joint may be advised to reduce the joint pain and restore the motion in the stiff and/or painful joints. Conditions such as osteoarthritis, tendonitis and post fracture stiffness are often treated with this technique.

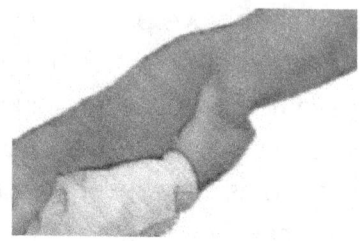

Deep Massage and Stretch

Massaging and stretching of the pectoralis group and scalene muscles are commonly advised to relieve muscle tightness. This helps in relaxing these muscles and reducing the tension over the nerves of the upper extremities.

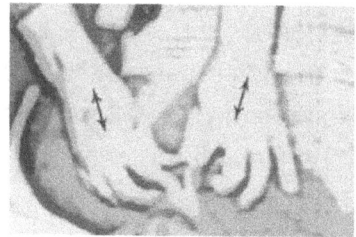

Neural Milking

Neural milking helps in the following ways. It restores normal neurophysiology and neuromechanics. It improves tension tolerance and intraneural and extraneural excursion. It improves vascular function and axoplasmic flow. Neural milking is performed by following the path of the nerve and applying gentle pressure. The median nerve is superficial medial to the biceps and indirectly at the carpal tunnel between the palmaris longus and flexor carpi radialis. The ulnar nerve is superficial at the pisiform area at the wrist and at the cubital tunnel between the olecranon and medial epicondyle. The radial nerve is most superficial at the mid humerus. The radial sensory nerve is most superficial on the lateral side of the forearm.

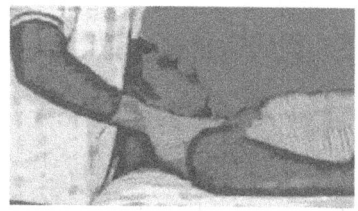

Stretch Tight Muscles

The suboccipital muscles are formed by the rectus capitis muscle and oblique capitis muscles. These muscles connect the central nervous system to the peripheral nervous system. If you have a tight suboccipital muscle, you have to take pressure off the nerves by stretching. This is achieved by positioning 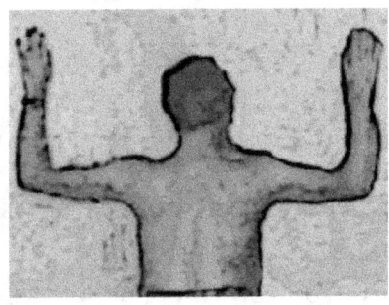 the patient in supine with the head resting in your hand. Then, gently pull in an upward direction. This maneuver stretches the suboccipital muscle group.

The scalene muscles have three bellies. When this muscle becomes tight, you will have an elevated shoulder girdle. To stretch the scalene muscles, position the patient in supine, side bend their head to the contralateral side and depress the shoulder girdle. You can add proprioceptive neuromuscular techniques or muscle energy techniques to increase the stretch.

To stretch the tight pectoralis muscle, stabilize the shoulder girdle and the glenohumeral joint. Then, pull the arm out into abduction. Poor posture or weak scapular stabilizers can cause tight pectoral muscles. The best way to stretch the pectoralis is to get close to a 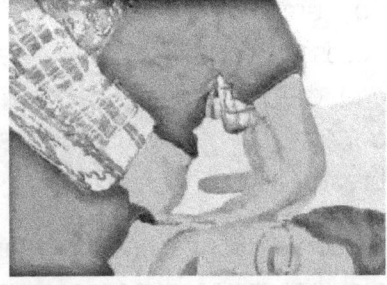 doorway, place your hands up against the doorway with the elbow flexed, then, step forward. Finally, move your body forward.

To stretch the upper trapezius, position the patient in supine with the head supported. Maximally flex the patient's head with simultaneous contralateral side flexion, and then rotate the chin toward the painful side. Add shoulder depression to increase the stretch.

For levator scapulae tightness, position the patient in supine. Maximally flex, contralaterally rotate and contralaterally flex the head. You may add contract and relax techniques to increase the stretch.

Poor posture can cause muscle imbalance. Tight muscles and weakened muscles can produce a vicious cycle of upper quadrant dysfunction. Aside from posture, there are physical complications that can add to this vicious cycle. These include factors such as smoking, weight problems, thyroid problems, fatigue, lack of sleep and decreased physical and mental fitness.

Stage III – Rehabilitative Processes

Rehabilitative processes are advised following reduction of symptoms. The restoration of the muscle shape and structure are important to relieve nerve tension. Rehabilitative processes enable the patients to resume work and prevent the recurrence of such events. Only over an extended period can adaptive tissue changes be corrected. During the subsequent periods, steps to increase overall aerobic capacity and fitness are advised. Consumption of a balanced diet and appropriate supplementation are also necessary for faster recovery and improved performance of the muscles and the nerve tissues. Postural corrections are to be re-emphasized during the rehabilitative process and so does the awareness about proper breathing techniques.

Nerve gliding or neurodynamics is a slow controlled movement. It is a movement-based management. You gently glide or mobilize a nerve, but you do not stretch the neural tissue. Start actively as opposed to passively so that your patients feel more comfortable. The nervous system adapts to body movement by gliding within the system. Nerve mobilization causes decreased intraneural and extraneural pressure. It also improves blood circulation. A slider is a non-aggressive movement that helps decrease anxiety in anxious patients. A tensioner is different from a slider because it is a more aggressive movement and it is pulling from both ends (Wright et al., 2005). Start with active movements followed by general slider and as progression goes along, then do the tensioner. Always test the non-involved extremity prior to testing the involved side (Pahor & Toppenberg, 1996; Coppieters et al., 2001; Lew & Briggs, 1997; Kerr, Vijnovich, & Bradnam, 2002).

CHAPTER 6

Review of Current Research and Concluding Remarks

Is nerve gliding an effective technique? The answer is YES. Kostopoulos et al. (2008) studied the differences in nerve conductivity of the tibial motor, peroneal motor, peroneal sensory, and sural nerves in patients with primary and secondary Raynaud's phenomenon. They conclude that the neural mobilization techniques can be applied to assist with patient symptoms. In another study, a patient with chronic lateral elbow pain who had signs of nerve entrapment was treated with neural mobilization techniques 14 times over a 10-week period. Ekstrom et al. (2002) noted that these techniques were successful in relieving the symptoms. The authors concluded that neural tension testing may be a useful examination procedure and mobilization may be a useful intervention for patients who have lateral elbow pain. Orset et al. (2000) noted that a 50 to 90% improvement was reported following neural mobilization in patients suffering from thoracic outlet syndrome. They conclude that utilization of peripheral nerve mobilization techniques to restore nerve gliding mobility could improve the results of conservative treatment. Authors Ellis and Hing (2008) evaluated the literature published about the efficacy of neural mobilization in the treatment of pathologies of the nervous system. Ten randomized clinical trials (discussed in eleven retrieved articles) were identified that discussed the therapeutic effect of neural mobilization. Although minimal, the use of neural mobilization has been supported. Further studies can shed light on the benefits of neural mobilization techniques (Ellis & Hing, 2008).

When using nerve mobilization techniques, start treating in the same position whether it is proximal to distal or distal to proximal. For an irritable disorder, treat remotely from the area of symptoms to get either proximal or distal gliding. For example, if somebody has median nerve entrapment distally at the wrist with painful wrist extension, treat at the elbow area and at the brachial plexus area. Passive mobilization techniques are applied in the available range of motion. Prescribe a home exercise program to maintain neural mobility. Upper limb tension testing allows you to differentiate between symptoms of local origin and symptoms arising from the nervous system (Butler, 1991).

Nerve mobilization can be accomplished with either the tensioner technique or the gliding technique. The tensioner technique can be quite painful when compared to the slider technique. Coppieters et al. (2009) sought to determine whether different types of nerve-gliding exercises are associated with different amounts of longitudinal nerve excursion. They used high-resolution ultrasound to measure longitudinal excursion of the median nerve in the upper arm during six different nerve-gliding exercises. They noted that different exercises induced different amounts of longitudinal nerve excursion. The "sliding technique" was associated with the largest excursion, while the amount of nerve movement associated with the "tensioning technique" was smaller than the nerve excursion induced with individual movements of the neck or elbow. The authors concluded that different types of neurodynamic techniques have different mechanical effects on the nervous system (Coppieters et al., 2009).

One should always assess the amount of active motion before initiating the passive ULTT. The passive motion can be evaluated using the ULTT. Pay close attention to encountered resistance and level of irritability. You should avoid progression beyond the end point of resistance and symptoms. The order of examination may be varied; however, the same order must be followed during subsequent examinations. Tender spots that may be contributing to the peripheral nerve must be evaluated within the cervical segment. Check for reproduction of symptoms or alteration in ROM; for example, in testing the median nerve, placing the wrist in neutral position increases elbow extension. The non-neural tissue should also be treated by placing nervous tissue in a slack for acute conditions.

Nerve gliding or neural mobilization is contraindicated for recently repaired peripheral nerve, malignancy, active inflammatory conditions, and demyelinating diseases. Adequate precautions should be followed to prevent worsening of irritable conditions such as spinal cord signs, nerve root signs, severe unremitting night pain lacking a diagnosis, recent paresthesia/anesthesia, and complex regional pain syndrome.

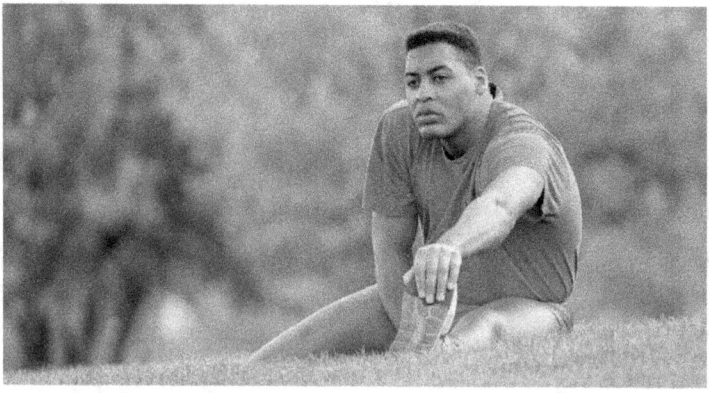

Successful implementation and relief from symptoms are achieved only when the treatment principles are correctly followed. Patient involvement is also very essential. It is necessary to educate the patient about factors such as source of symptoms, contributing factors, precautions, and contraindications. This helps in better patient compliance. The home programs must be diligently followed by the patients for faster recovery and prevention of the symptoms. One should also remember to place tension at the nerve at a remote site. Although it is unlikely to improve the internal structure of the nerve, nerve mobilization improves the nerve's ability to glide within the tissue bed. Lastly, there are no clear guidelines or research that supports the most effective amplitude, dosage, or duration of nerve gliding procedure. The procedures must be individualized according to the needs of the specific patient.

References

Barr, A. E., & Barbe, M. F. (2002). Pathophysiological tissue changes associated with repetitive movement: A review of the evidence. Physical Therapy, 82(2), 173–187. Retrieved from ptjournal.apta.org/content/82/2/173.full

Bove, G. (2008). Epi-Perineurial anatomy, innervation, and axonal nociceptive mechanisms. Journal of bodywork and movement therapies, 12(3), 185–190. Retrieved from http://www.ncbi.nlm.nih.gov/pmc/articles/PMC2610338/

Butler, D. S. (2000). The sensitive nervous system. Adelaide, Australia: Noigroup Publications.

Butler, D. S., & Jones, M. A. (1991). Mobilisation of the nervous system. City: Elsevier Health Sciences.

Butler, D., & Gifford, L. (1989). The concept of adverse mechanical tension in nervous system. Part 1: Testing for dural tension. Physiotherapy, 75(1), 623–636. Retrieved from www.jospt.org/members/getfile.asp?id=1354

Calvin, W. H., Devor, M., & Howe, J. F. (1982). Can neuralgias arise from minor demyelination? Spontaneous firing, mechanosensitivity, and after-discharge from conducting axons. Experimental Neurology, 75(1), 755–763. Retrieved from http://williamcalvin.com/1980s/1982ExpNeurol.pdf

Chen, A. C. (2008). Pain perception and its genesis in the human brain. Sheng Li Xue Bao, 60(5), 677–85. Retrieved from http://www.actaps.com.cn/qikan/manage/wenzhang/2008-5-17.pdf

Coppieters, M. W., & Butler, D. S. (2008). Do 'sliders' slide and 'tensioners' tension? An analysis of neurodynamic techniques and considerations regarding their application. Manual Therapy, 13(3), 21–1. Retrieved from

http://www.theforgottenjoint.com/wp-content/uploads/2011/02/neural.
pdf

Coppieters, M. W., Hough, A. D., & Dilley, A. (2009). Different nerve-gliding exercises induce different magnitudes of median nerve longitudinal excursion: An in vivo study using dynamic ultrasound imaging. Journal of Orthopaedic & Sports Physical Therapy, 39(3),164–71. Retrieved from www.jospt.org/issues/articleID.2276,type.2/article_detail.asp

Coppieters, M. W., Stappaerts, K. H., Everaert, D. G., & Staes, F. F. (2001). Addition of test components during neurodynamic testing: Effect on range of motion and sensory responses. Journal of Orthopaedic & Sports Physical Therapy, 31(5), 226–35. Retrieved from www.jospt.org/issues/articleID.353,type.14/article_detail.asp

D'Mello, R., & Dickenson, A. H. (2008). Spinal cord mechanisms of pain. British journal of anaesthesia, 101(1), 8–16. doi: 10.1093/bja/aen088

Davis, D. S., Anderson, I. B., Carson, M. G., Elkins, C. L., & Stuckey, L. B. (2008). Upper limb neural tension and seated slump tests: The false positive rate among healthy young adults without cervical or lumbar symptoms. Journal of Manual and Manipulative Therapy, 16(3),136– 41. Retrieved from http://www.ncbi.nlm.nih.gov/pmc/articles/PMC2582423/

Eaton, C. (2007). Nerve injury classification. Available from http://www.eatonhand.com/clf/clf310.htm

Ekstrom, R. A., & Holden, K. (2002). Examination of and intervention for a patient with chronic lateral elbow pain with signs of nerve entrapment. Physical Therapy, 82(11), 1077–86. Retrieved from ptjournal.apta.org/content/82/11/1077.full

Ellis, R. F., & Hing, W. A. (2008). Neural mobilization: A systematic review of randomized controlled trials with an analysis of therapeutic efficacy. Journal of Manual and Manipulative Therapy 2008, 16(1), 8–22.

Elvey, R. (1986). Treatment of arm pain associated with abnormal brachial plexus tension. Australian Journal of Physiotherapy , 32(4), 225–230.

Gelberman, R. H., Yamaguchi, K., Hollstien, S. B., Winn, S.S., Heidenreich, F.P. Jr., Bindra, R.R., Hsieh, P., Silva, M.J. (1998). Changes in interstitial pressure and cross-sectional area of the cubital tunnel and of the ulnar nerve with flexion of the elbow: An experimental study in human cadavera. The Journal of Bone & Joint Surgery, 80(4), 492–501.

Kerr, J. M., Vujnovich, A. L., & Bradnam, L. (2002). Changes in alpha-motoneuron excitability with positions that tension neural tissue. Electromyography & Clinical Neurophysiology, 42(8), 459–71.

Kleinrensink, G. J., Stoeckart, R., Mulder, P. G., Hoek, G., Broek, T., Vleeming, A., & Snijders, C. J. (2000). Upper limb tension tests as tools in the diagnosis of nerve and plexus lesions: Anatomical and biomechanical aspects. Clinical biomechanics (Bristol, Avon), 15(1), 9–14.

Kostopoulos, D., Rizopoulos, K., & Vartholomeos, N. (2008). Nerve conduction velocities in the lower extremity in patients with Raynaud's phenomenon and clinical applications. Journal of bodywork and movement therapies, 12(1), 58–66. Retrieved from www.handsonseminars.com/RAYNAUD.pdf

Lew, P. C., & Briggs, C. A. (1997). Relationship between the cervical component of the slump test and change in hamstring muscle tension. Manual Therapy, 2(2), 98–105. doi: 10.1054/math.1997.0291

Mackinnon, S. E. (2002). Pathophysiology of nerve compression. Hand clinics, 18(2),231– 41.

Magee, D. (2002). Orthopedic physical assessment (4th ed.). Philadelphia: Saunders.

Maitland, G. (1985). The slump test: Examination and treatment. Australian Journal of Physiotherapy, 31(1), 215–219.

Maitland, G. D. (1979). Negative disc exploration: Positive canal signs. Australian Journal of Physiotherapy, 25(3), 129–134. Retrieved from http://ajp.physiotherapy.asn.au/AJP/vol_25/3/AustJPhysiotherv25i3Maitland.pdf

Maitland, G. D. (1980). Movement of pain sensitive structures in the vertebral canal and intervertebral foramina in a group of group of Physiotherapy students. South African Journal of Physiotherapy, 36(1) 4–12.

Marchettini, P., Lacerenza, M., Mauri, E., & Marangoni, C. (2006). Painful peripheral neuropathies. Current Neuropharmacology, 4(3),175–81. Retrieved from http://www.ncbi.nlm.nih.gov/pmc/articles/PMC2430688/

Messlinger, K. (1997). What is a nociceptor? Der Anaesthesist, 46(2),142–53.

Millesi, H., Zöch, G., & Rath, T. (1998). The gliding apparatus of peripheral nerve and its clinical significance. Journal of Orthopaedic & Sports Physical Therapy, 27(1),16–21.

O'Neill, P. J., Parks, B. G., Walsh, R., Simmons, L. M., & Miller, S. D. (2007). Excursion and strain of the superficial peroneal nerve during inversion ankle sprain. The Journal of Bone & Joint Surgery, 89(5), 979–986.

O'Driscoll, S. W., Horii, E., Carmichael, S. W., Morrey BF (1991). The cubital tunnel and ulnar neuropathy. The Journal of bone and joint surgery. British volume, 73(4):613-7. Retrieved from http://www.bjj.boneandjoint.org.uk/content/73-B/4/613.long

Orset, G. (2000). Evaluation of the cervicothoracobrachial outlet and results of conservative treatment Chirurgie de la main, 19(4), 212–7.

Pahor, S., & Toppenberg, R. (1996). An investigation of neural tissue involvement in ankle inversion sprains. Manual Therapy, 1(4), 192–197.

Rigoard, P., & Lapierre, F. (2009). Review of the peripheral nerve. Neurochirurgie. Advance online publication. doi:10.1136/jnnp.14.2.76

Robinson, D. R., & Gebhart, G. F. (2008). Inside information: The unique features of visceral sensation. Molecular interventions, 8(5), 242–53. doi: 10.1124/mi.8.5.9

Rozmaryn, L. M., Dovelle, S., Rothman, E. R., Gorman, K., Olvey, K. M., Bartko, J. J. (1998). Nerve and tendon gliding exercises and the conservative management of carpal tunnel syndrome. Journal of hand therapy : official journal of the American Society of Hand, 11(3), 171–9.

Rubinstein, S. M., & van Tulder, M. (2008). A best-evidence review of diagnostic procedures for neck and low-back pain. Best practice & research. Clinical rheumatology, 22(3),471– 82. doi: 10.1016/j.berh.2007.12.003

Seddon, H. J. (1942). A classification of nerve injuries. British Medical Journal, 7(2), 560–561. Retrieved from http://www.ncbi.nlm.nih.gov/pmc/articles/PMC2164563/pdf/brmedj04015-0028c.pdf

Shacklock, M. (2005). Clinical neurodynamics: A new system of musculoskeletal treatment. Sydney, Australia: Elsevier Butterworth Heinemann.

Shacklock, M. O. (1995). Neurodynamics. Physiotherapy, 81, 9–16.

Stevens, J. H. (1934). Brachial plexus paralysis. In E. A. Codman (Ed.) The shoulder (pp. 344–350). Boston: Privately Published.

Sunderland, S (1951). A classification of peripheral nerve injuries producing loss of function. Brain, 74(4), 491–516.

Sunderland, S. (1965). The connective tissues of the peripheral nerves. Brain, 88(4), 841–54.

Sunderland, S. (1978). Nerve and nerve injuries (2nd ed.). New York: Churchill Livingstone.

Topp, K. S., & Boyd, B. S. (2006). Structure and biomechanics of peripheral nerves: Nerve responses to physical stresses and implications for physical therapist practice. Physical Therapy, 86(1), 92–109. Retrieved from ptjournal.apta.org/content/86/1/92.full

Turl, S. E., & George, K. P. (1998). Adverse neural tension: A factor in repetitive hamstring strain? Journal of Orthopaedic & Sports Physical Therapy, 27(1),16–21. Retrieved from www.jospt.org/members/getfile.asp?id=817

Walsh, M. T. (2005). Upper limb neural tension testing and mobilization: Fact, fiction, and a practical approach. Journal of hand therapy: official journal of the American Society of Hand, 18(2), 241–258. doi: 10.1197/j. jht.2005.02.010

Walsh, M. T. Rationale and indications for the use of nerve mobilization and nerve gliding as a treatment approach. In J. M. Hunter, E. J. Mackin, & A. D. Callahan (Eds.) Rehabilitation of the hand and upper extremity (5th ed., pp. 762–75). Philadelphia: Mosby.

Wilgis, E. F., & Murphy, R. (1986). The significance of longitudinal excursion in peripheral nerves. Hand clinics, 2(4), 761–766.

Wright, T. W., Glowczewskie, F., Cowin, D., & Wheeler, D. L. (2005). Radial nerve excursion and strain at the elbow and wrist associated with upper-extremity motion. The Journal of hand surgery, 30(5), 990–6. doi: 10.1016/j. jhsa.2005.06.008

Wright, T. W., Glowczewskie, F., Cowin, D., & Wheeler, D. L. (2005). Radial nerve excursion and strain at the elbow and wrist associated with upper-extremity motion. The Journal of hand surgery, 30(5),990–6. doi: 10.1016/j. jhsa.2005.06.008

APPENDIX

Examination

Upon meeting the Satisfactory Completion Statement, you may receive a certificate of completion at the end of this course.

Contact ceu@rehabsurge.com to find out if this distance learning course is an approved course from your board. Save your course outline and contact your own board or organization for specific filing requirements.

In order to obtain continuing education hours, you must have read the book, have completed the exam and survey. Please include a $10.00 exam fee to process your exam. Mail the exam answer sheet and survey sheet to:

CEU certificate request
Rehabsurge, Inc.
PO Box 287
Baldwin, NY 11510

Allow 2-4 weeks to receive your certificate.

You can also take the exam online at www.rehabsurge.com. Register and pay the exam fee of $10.00. Once, you have passed the exam with the score of 70%, you will be able to print your certificate immediately. See rehabsurge.com for more details.

Exam Questions

1. Which nerve connective tissue layer forms the initial covering of the nerve fibers after the myelin sheath?

   a. epineurium

   b. perineurium

   c. endoneurium

   d. paraneurium

2. What is the science of the relationship between the mechanics and physiology of the nervous system?

   a. neurology

   b. neurodynamics

   c. neurophysiology

   d. neuromechanics

3. In a study done by Wright and colleagues, how many cm does the median nerve slide at the wrist from wrist extension to wrist flexion?

   a. 1

   b. 2

   c. 3

   d. 4

4. O' Driscoll determined that the cubital tunnel is smaller during flexion by how many percentage points compared to extension?

   a. 25%

   b. 50%

   c. 75%

   d. 100%

5. What is the term for a condition where pain is felt from stimuli that does not hurt in normal circumstances?

   a. anesthesia

   b. hyperpathia

   c. allodynia

   d. hypoesthesia

6. Which type of nerve injury is described as a physiologic block of the nerve; with demyelination of the nerve at the site of injury?

   a. neuropraxia; Sunderland I

   b. axonotmesis; Sunderland II

   c. axonotmesis; Sunderland III

   d. neurotmesis; Sunderland V

7. Which type of neural tension test is performed by stabilizing the pelvis, flexing the head and moving a limb?

   a. slump test

   b. straight leg raise

   c. Elvey test

   d. upper limb tension test

8. The upper limb tension test is considered positive except for:

   a. reproduction of symptoms

   b. different symptoms from the left and right

   c. tingling and numbness

   d. alteration in range

9. Which upper limb tension test requires elbow flexion?

    a. Radial

    b. Median

    c. Ulnar

    d. Musculocutaneous

10. You have your patient flex the elbow at 90 degrees; then, fully supinate at the forearm. You ask the patient to resist coming into pronation. You are testing median nerve entrapment at the:

    a. pronator teres

    b. fibrous band and lacertus fibrosus

    c. fibrous arch of the flexor digitorum superficialis

    d. carpal tunnel

11. If you hold a piece of paper, instead of adducting, you substitute with flexion of the thumb interphalangeal joint. This is called:

    a. Egawa's sign

    b. Wartenburg's sign

    c. Froment's sign

    d. Jeanne's sign

12. All of the following exercises can improve gliding of the median nerve except:

    a. Balloon patting

    b. Alphabet letters

    c. Crawling exercises

    d. Plate carrying

13. The following are techniques you can use for Stage I-symptom control except for:

    a. behavior modification

    b. workplace modification

    c. improve breathing pattern

    d. muscle stripping

14. Which technique is performed by following the path of the nerve and applying gentle pressure?

    a. muscle stripping

    b. neural milking

    c. joint mobilization

    d. effleurage

15. Which muscle are you stretching when you position the patient in supine; side bend the head and depress the shoulder girdle?

    a. suboccipital muscles

    b. scalene muscles

    c. pectoralis muscles

    d. upper trapezius

16. Which type of nerve mobilization technique is aggressive and requires pulling from both ends of the nerve?

    a. slider

    b. tensioner

    c. flossing

    d. gliding

17. If a patient complains of acute carpal tunnel syndrome, which movement should you avoid when performing nerve gliding?

   a. elbow extension

   b. wrist extension

   c. forearm supination

   d. shoulder depression

18. Ekstrom et al treated a patient with chronic lateral elbow pain who had signs of nerve entrapment. What is the frequency of their treatment?

   a. times over a 10 week period

   b. 10 times over a 10 week period

   c. 14 times over a 6 week period

   d. 10 times over a 6 week period

19. When performing nerve mobilization techniques, which type of motion should you perform initially?

   a. active

   b. active-assistive

   c. passive

   d. resistive

20. Nerve mobilization is contraindicated in all of the following conditions except for:

   a. recently repaired peripheral nerve

   b. complex regional pain syndrome

   c. malignancy

   d. active inflammatory condition

Answer Sheet

Name: _____

Address: _____

Profession: _____

License Number: _____

Date: _____

E-mail Address (optional): _____

Exam:

1. a b c d	11. a b c d
2. a b c d	12. a b c d
3. a b c d	13. a b c d
4. a b c d	14. a b c d
5. a b c d	15. a b c d
6. a b c d	16. a b c d
7. a b c d	17. a b c d
8. a b c d	18. a b c d
9. a b c d	19. a b c d
10. a b c d	20. a b c d

Please mail $10.00 and completed form to:

CEU certificate request

Rehabsurge, Inc.
PO Box 287, Baldwin, NY 11510.
Phone: +1 (516) 515-1267
Email: ceu@rehabsurge.com

Alternatively, you can take the exam online at www.rehabsurge.com. You will receive your certificate instantly.

It is the learner's responsibility to comply with all state and national regulatory board's rules and regulations. This includes but is not limited to:

- verifying and complying with applicable continuing education requirements;
- verifying and complying with all applicable standards of practice;
- verifying and complying with all licensure requirements;
- any other rules or laws identified in the learners state or regulatory board that is not mentioned here.

It is the learner's responsibility to complete ALL coursework in order to receive credit. This includes but is not limited to:

- Reading all course materials fully;
- Completing all course activities to meet the criteria set forth by the instructor;
- Completing and passing all applicable tests and quizzes. All learner's MUST take a comprehensive online exam where they MUST get at least 70%. Getting 70% is a requirement to pass.

IMPORTANT: Rehabsurge reserves the right to deny continuing education credits or withdraw credits issued at any time if: Coursework is found to be incomplete; It is determined that a user falsified, copied, and/or engaged in any flagrant attempt to manipulate, modify, or alter the coursework just to receive credit; and/or It is determined that the coursework was not completed by the user.

If any of the conditions above are determined, Rehabsurge reserves the right to notify any applicable state and national boards along with supporting documentation.

Program Evaluation Form

Rehabsurge, Inc. works to develop new programs based on your comments and suggestions, making your feedback on the program very important to us. We would appreciate you taking a few moments to evaluate this program.

Course Start Date:_____ Course End Date: _____

Course Start Time:_____ Course End Time:_____

Identity Verification: Name:_____

Profession:_____

License Number:_____

State: _____

Please initial to indicate that you are the individual who read the book and completed the test. Initial here:_____

May we use your comments and suggestions in upcoming marketing materials?   Yes   No

Would you take another seminar from Rehabsurge, Inc.?   Yes   No

The educational level required to read the book is:

	Beginner	Intermediate	Advanced

The course is:	(5-Yes/Excellent)	(1-No/Poor)		
Relevant to my profession	5	4	3	2	1
Valuable to my profession	5	4	3	2	1
Content matched stated objectives	5	4	3	2	1
Complete coverage of materials	5	4	3	2	1
Teaching ability	5	4	3	2	1
Organization of material	5	4	3	2	1
Effective	5	4	3	2	1

Please rate the objectives. After reading the material, how well do you feel you are able to meet?

Objective 1	5	4	3	2	1
Objective 2	5	4	3	2	1
Objective 3	5	4	3	2	1
Objective 4	5	4	3	2	1
Objective 5	5	4	3	2	1

What was the most beneficial part of the program? What was the least beneficial part of the program? _____

_____

_____

_____

What would you like to see added to the program? In what ways might we make this program experience better for you?_____

_____

_____

_____

If you have any general comments on this topic or program please explain.

_____

_____

_____

_____

Please tell us what other programs or topics might interest you?

_____

_____

_____

_____

Thank you for participating and taking the time to join us today!

www.ingramcontent.com/pod-product-compliance
Lightning Source LLC
Chambersburg PA
CBHW081220170526
45165CB00009B/2882